THE DEFINITIVE PLANT BASED DIET COOKBOOK FOR BEGINNERS

Easy and affordable recipes that beginners and advanced can cook on a budget. Regain confidence and lose weight fast

Ursa Males

TABLE OF CONTENTS

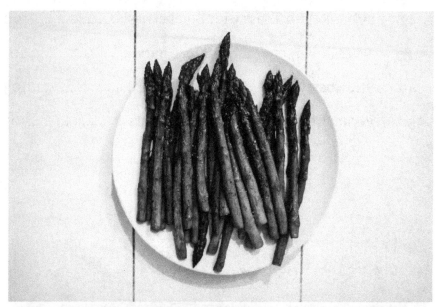

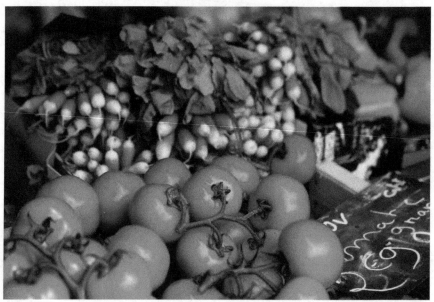

BREAKFAST

1. Vegan Breakfast Biscuits

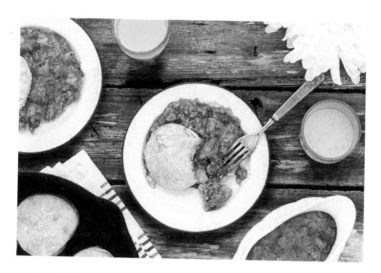

Preparation Time: 10 minutes

Cooking Time: 10 min

Servings: 6

Ingredients:

- 2 cups Almond Flour
- 1 tbsp Baking Powder
- ¼ teaspoon Salt
- ½ teaspoon Onion Powder
- ½ cup Coconut Milk
- ¼ cup Nutritional Yeast

- 2 tbsp Ground Flax Seeds
- ¼ cup Olive Oil

Directions:

1. Preheat oven to 450°F. Whisk together all ingredients in a bowl. Divide the batter into a pre-greased muffin tin. Bake for 10 minutes.

Nutrition: Calories: 432 Fat: 5g Carbs: 13g Protein: 8g

2. **Orange French Toast**

Preparation Time: 5 minutes

Cooking Time: 30 minutes

Servings: 8 servings

Ingredients:

- 2 cups of plant milk (unflavored)
- 4 tablespoon maple syrup
- 11/2 tablespoon cinnamon
- Salt (optional)
- 1 cup flour (almond)
- 1 tablespoon orange zest
- 8 bread slices

Directions:

1. Turn the oven and heat to 400°F afterward. In a cup, add ingredients and whisk until the batter is smooth.
2. Dip each piece of bread into the paste and permit to soak for a couple of seconds. Put in the pan, and cook until lightly browned.
3. Put the toast on the cookie sheet and bake for ten to fifteen minutes in the oven until it is crispy.

Nutrition: Calories: 129 Fat: 1.1g Carbs: 21.5g Protein: 7.9g

3. Chocolate Chip Coconut Pancakes

Preparation Time: 5 minutes

Cooking Time: 30 minutes

Servings: 8 servings

Ingredients:

- 11/4 cup oats
- 2 teaspoons coconut flakes
- 2 cup plant milk
- 11/4 cup maple syrup
- 11/3 cup of chocolate chips
- 2 1/4 cups buckwheat flour
- 2 teaspoon baking powder
- 1 teaspoon vanilla essence
- 2 teaspoon flaxseed meal
- Salt (optional)

Directions:

1. Put the flaxseed and cook over medium heat until the paste becomes a little moist. Remove seeds. Stir the buckwheat, oats, coconut chips, baking powder, and salt with each other in a wide dish.

2. In a large dish, stir together the retained flax water with the sugar, maple syrup, vanilla essence. Transfer

the wet fixings to the dry ingredients and shake to combine.

3. Place over medium heat the nonstick grill pan. Pour 1/4 cup flour onto the grill pan with each pancake, and scatter gently. Cook for five to six minutes before the pancakes appear somewhat crispy.

Nutrition: Calories: 198 Fat: 9.1g Carbs: 11.5g Protein: 7.9g

4. <u>**Apple-Lemon Bowl**</u>

Preparation time: 15 minutes

Cooking time: 0 minutes

Servings: 1-2

Ingredients:

- 6 apples
- 3 tablespoons walnuts
- 7 dates
- Lemon juice
- 1/2 teaspoon cinnamon

Directions:

1. Root the apples, then break them into wide bits. In a food cup, put seeds, part of the lime juice, almonds, spices, and three-quarters of the apples.
2. Thinly slice until finely ground. Apply the remaining apples and lemon juice and make slices.

Nutrition: Calories: 249 Fat: 5.1g Carbohydrates: 71.5g Protein: 7.9g

5. Black Bean and Sweet Potato Hash

Preparation time: 10 minutes

Cooking time: 14 minutes

Servings: 4

Ingredients:

- 1 cup onion (chopped)
- 1/3 cup vegetable broth
- 2 garlic (minced)
- 1 cup cooked black beans
- 2 teaspoons hot chili powder
- 2 cups chopped sweet potatoes

Directions:

1. Put the onions in a saucepan over medium heat and add the seasoning, and mix.
2. Add potatoes and chili flakes, then mix.
3. Cook for around 12 minutes more until the vegetables are cooked thoroughly.
4. Add the green onion, beans, and salt.

5.

6. Cook for more than 2 minutes and serve.

Nutrition: Calories: 239 Fat: 1.1g Carbohydrates: 71.5g Protein: 7.9g

6. <u>Apple-Walnut Breakfast Bread</u>

Preparation time: 15 minutes

Cooking time: 25 minutes

Servings: 8

Ingredients:

- 11/2 cups apple sauce
- 1/3 cup plant milk
- 2 cups all-purpose flour
- Salt to taste
- 1 teaspoon ground cinnamon
- 1 tablespoon flax seeds mixed with 2 tablespoons warm water
- 3/4 cup brown sugar
- 1 teaspoon baking powder
- 1/2 cup chopped walnuts

Directions:

1. Preheat to 375 degrees Fahrenheit. Combine the apple sauce, sugar, milk, and flax mixture in a jar and mix. Combine the flour, baking powder, salt, and cinnamon in a separate bowl.
2. Simply add dry Ingredients: into the wet fixings and combine to make slices.

3. Bake for 25 minutes until it becomes light brown.

Nutrition: Calories: 309 Fat: 9.1g Carbohydrates: 16.5g
Protein: 6.9g

7. <u>Mint Chocolate Green Protein Smoothie</u>

Preparation time: 5 minutes

Cooking time: 0 minutes

Servings: 1

Ingredients:

- 1 scoop chocolate powder
- 1 tablespoon flaxseed
- 1 banana
- 1 mint leaf
- 3/4 cup almond milk
- 3 tablespoons dark chocolate (chopped)

Directions:

1. Blend all the fixings except the dark chocolate. Garnish dark chocolate when ready.

Nutrition: Calories: 115 Carbs: 22g Fat: 2g Protein: 6g

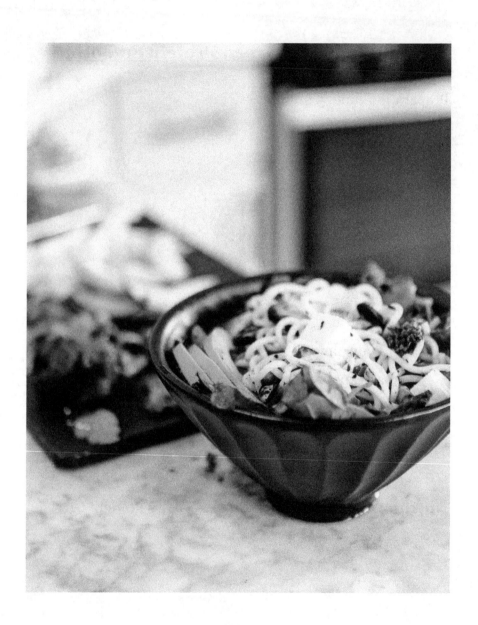

LUNCH

8. Cauliflower and Artichokes Soup

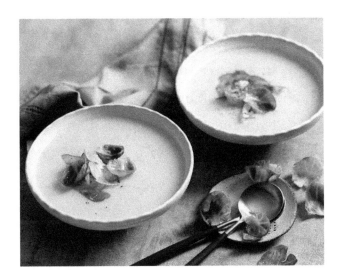

Preparation time: 10 minutes

Cooking time: 25 minutes

Servings: 4

Ingredients:

- 1 pound cauliflower florets
- 1 cup canned artichoke hearts, drained & chopped
- 2 scallions, chopped
- 2 tablespoons olive oil
- 2 garlic cloves, minced
- 6 cups vegetable stock

- Salt and black pepper to the taste
- 2/3 cup coconut cream
- 2 tablespoons cilantro, chopped

Directions:

1. Heat-up a pot with the oil over medium heat, add the scallions and the garlic, and sauté for 5 minutes.
2. Add the cauliflower and the other fixings, toss, bring to a simmer and cook over medium heat for 20 minutes more. Blend the soup using an immersion blender, divide it into bowls and serve.

Nutrition: Calories 207Fat 17.2gCarbs 14.1gProtein 4.7g

9. Hot Cabbage Soup

Preparation time: 10 minutes

Cooking time: 30 minutes

Servings: 4

Ingredients:

- 3 spring onions, chopped
- 1 green cabbage head, shredded
- 2 tablespoons olive oil
- 1 tablespoon ginger, grated
- 1 teaspoon cumin, ground
- 6 cups vegetable stock
- Salt and black pepper to the taste
- 1 teaspoon hot paprika
- 1 teaspoon chili powder
- 1 tablespoon cilantro, chopped

Directions:

1. Heat-up your pot with the oil over medium heat, add the spring onions, ginger, and the cumin, and sauté for 5 minutes.
2. Add the cabbage and the other ingredients, stir, bring to a simmer and cook over medium heat for 25 minutes more.

3. Ladle the soup into bowls and serve for lunch.

Nutrition: Calories 117Fat 7.5gCarbs 12.7gProtein 2.8g

10. **Classic Black Beans Chili**

Preparation time: 10 minutes

Cooking time: 3 hours

Servings: 4

Ingredients:

- ½ cup quinoa
- 2 and ½ cups veggie stock
- 14 ounces canned tomatoes, chopped
- 15 ounces canned black beans, drained
- ¼ cup green bell pepper, chopped
- ¼ cup red bell pepper, chopped
- A pinch of salt and black pepper
- 2 garlic cloves, minced
- 1 carrot, shredded
- 1 small chili pepper, chopped
- 2 teaspoons chili powder
- 1 teaspoon cumin, ground
- A pinch of cayenne pepper
- ½ cup of corn
- 1 teaspoon oregano, dried

For the vegan sour cream:

- A drizzle of apple cider vinegar
- 4 tablespoons water

- ½ cup cashews, soaked overnight and drained
- 1 teaspoon lime juice

Directions:

1. Put the stock in your slow cooker. Add quinoa, tomatoes, beans, red and green bell pepper, garlic, carrot, salt, pepper, corn, cumin, cayenne, chili powder, chili pepper oregano, stir, cover, and cook on high for 3 hours.

2. Meanwhile, put the cashews in your blender. Add water, vinegar, and lime juice and pulse well. Divide beans chili into bowls, top with vegan sour cream, and serve.

Nutrition: Calories 300Fat 4gCarbs 10gProtein 7g

11. <u>Amazing Potato Dish</u>

Preparation time: 10 minutes

Cooking time: 3 hours

Servings: 4

Ingredients:

- 1 and ½ pounds potatoes, peeled and roughly chopped
- 1 tablespoon olive oil
- 3 tablespoons water
- 1 small yellow onion, chopped
- ½ cup veggie stock cube, crumbled
- ½ teaspoon coriander, ground
- ½ teaspoon cumin, ground
- ½ teaspoon garam masala
- ½ teaspoon chili powder
- Black pepper to the taste
- ½ pound spinach, roughly torn

Directions:

1. Put the potatoes in your slow cooker. Add oil, water, onion, stock cube, coriander, cumin, garam masala, chili powder, black pepper, and spinach.
2. Stir, cover, and cook on high within 3 hours.
3. Divide into bowls and serve. Enjoy!

Nutrition: Calories 270Fat 4gCarbs 8gProtein 12g

12. Sweet Potatoes and Lentils Delight

Preparation time: 10 minutes

Cooking time: 4 hours and 30 minutes

Servings: 6

Ingredients:

- 6 cups sweet potatoes, peeled and cubed
- 2 teaspoons coriander, ground
- 2 teaspoons chili powder
- 1 yellow onion, chopped
- 3 cups veggie stock
- 4 garlic cloves, minced
- A pinch of sea salt
- black pepper
- 10 ounces canned coconut milk
- 1 cup of water
- 1 and ½ cups red lentils

Directions:

1. Put sweet potatoes in your slow cooker. Add coriander, chili powder, onion, stock, garlic, salt, and pepper, stir, cover and cook on high for 3 hours.
2. Add lentils, stir, cover, and cook for 1 hour and 30 minutes.

3. Add water and coconut milk, stir well, divide into bowls, and serve right away. Enjoy!

Nutrition Calories 300 Fat 10g Carbs 16g Protein 10g

13. **Mushroom Stew**

Preparation time: 10 minutes

Cooking time: 8 hours

Servings: 4

Ingredients:

- 2 garlic cloves, minced
- 1 celery stalk, chopped
- 1 yellow onion, chopped
- 1 and ½ cups firm tofu, pressed and cubed
- 1 cup of water
- 10 ounces mushrooms, chopped
- 1-pound mixed peas, corn, and carrots
- 2 and ½ cups veggie stock
- 1 teaspoon thyme, dried
- 2 tablespoons coconut flour
- A pinch of sea salt
- Black pepper to the taste

Directions:

1. Put the water and stock in your slow cooker. Add garlic, onion, celery, mushrooms, mixed veggies, tofu, thyme, salt, pepper, and flour.
2. Stir everything, cover, and cook on low for 8 hours. Divide into bowls and serve hot.

3. Enjoy!

Nutrition: Calories 230 Fat 4g Carbs 10g Protein 7g

14. **Simple Tofu Dish**

Preparation time: 10 minutes

Cooking time: 3 hours

Servings: 6

Ingredients:

- 1 big tofu package, cubed
- 1 tablespoon sesame oil
- ¼ cup pineapple, cubed
- 1 tablespoon olive oil
- 2 garlic cloves, minced
- 1 tablespoon brown rice vinegar
- 2 teaspoon ginger, grated
- ¼ cup soy sauce
- 5 big zucchinis, cubed
- ¼ cup sesame seeds

Directions:

1. In your food processor, mix sesame oil with pineapple, olive oil, garlic, ginger, soy sauce, and vinegar and whisk well.
2. Add this to your slow cooker and mix with tofu cubes. Cover and cook on High within 2 hours and 45 minutes.

3. Add sesame seeds and zucchinis, stir gently, cover, and cook on High for 15 minutes. Divide between plates and serve. Enjoy!

Nutrition: Calories 200 Fat 3gCarbs 9g Protein 10g

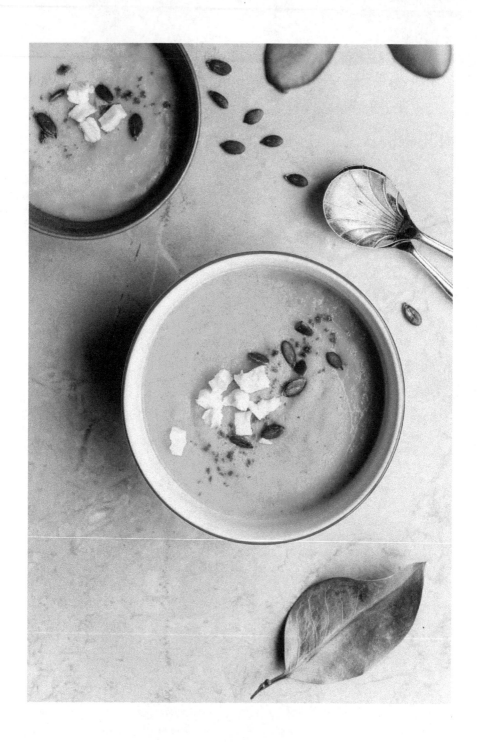

15. Chickpeas & Sweet Potato Curry

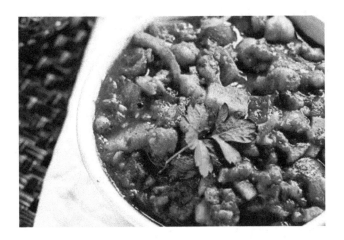

Preparation time: 15 minutes

Cooking time: 55 minutes

Servings: 2

Ingredients:

- 1 teaspoon olive oil
- 1 small onion, chopped
- 2 garlic cloves, chopped finely
- 2 cups tomatoes, chopped finely
- 1 teaspoon curry powder
- ½ teaspoon red chili powder
- Salt and ground black pepper, to taste

- 1 small sweet potato, peeled and cubed
- 1 (14-ounce) can chickpeas, drained and rinsed
- 7 ounces full-fat coconut milk

Directions:

1. Heat-up olive oil in a saucepan over medium heat and sauté the onion and garlic for about 4–5 minutes.
2. Add the tomatoes, spices, salt, and black pepper, and cook for about 2–3 minutes, crushing the tomatoes with the back of spoon.
3. Stir in the sweet potato and cook for about 1–2 minutes. Mix in the chickpeas plus coconut milk and bring to a boil over high heat.
4. Now, adjust the heat to medium-low and simmer, partially covered for about 35–40 minutes. Serve hot.

Nutrition: Calories 480 Fat 23.8 g Carbs 547 g Protein 13.8 g

16. <u>Beans & Mushroom Chili</u>

Preparation time: 15 minutes

Cooking time: 1 hour & 25 minutes

Servings: 4

Ingredients:

- 2 tablespoons avocado oil
- 1 medium onion, chopped
- 1 carrot, peeled and chopped
- 1 small bell pepper, seeded, and chopped
- 1-pound fresh mushrooms, sliced
- 2 garlic cloves, minced
- 2 teaspoons dried oregano
- 1 tablespoon red chili powder
- 1 tablespoon ground cumin
- Salt and ground black pepper, to taste
- 8 ounces 1 canned red kidney beans, rinsed & drained
- 8 ounces canned white kidney beans, rinsed and drained
- 2 cups tomatoes, chopped finely
- 1½ cups vegetable broth

Directions:

1. Heat-up the oil in a large Dutch oven over medium-low heat and cook the onions, carrot and bell pepper for about 10 minutes, stirring frequently.

2. Now, adjust the heat to medium-high. Stir in the mushrooms plus garlic and cook for about 5–6 minutes, stirring frequently.

3. Add the oregano, spices, salt, and black pepper, and cook for about chili 1–2 minutes. Stir in the beans, tomatoes, and broth, and bring to a boil.

4. Now, adjust the heat to low and simmer, covered for about 1 hour, stirring occasionally. Serve hot.

Nutrition: Calories 293 Fat 2.2 g Carbs 89 g Protein 28.5 g

17.   **Teriyaki Tofu with Broccoli**

Preparation time: 15 minutes

Cooking time: 25 minutes

Servings: 3

Ingredients:

Tofu:

- 14 ounces firm tofu, drained, pressed, and cut into 1-inch slices
- 1/3 cup cornstarch, divided
- 1/3 cup olive oil
- 1 teaspoon fresh ginger, grated
- 1 medium onion, sliced thinly
- 3 tablespoons low-sodium soy sauce
- 2 tablespoons balsamic vinegar
- 1 tablespoon maple syrup
- 1 teaspoon sesame oil
- ½ cup water

Steamed Broccoli:

- 2 cups broccoli florets

Directions:

1. In a shallow bowl, place ¼ cup of the cornstarch. Add the tofu cubes and coat with cornstarch.

2. In a cast iron skillet, heat the olive oil over medium heat and cook the tofu cubes for about 8–10 minutes or until golden from all sides.

3. With a slotted spoon, transfer the tofu cubes onto a plate. Set aside. Put the ginger in the same skillet, and sauté for about 1 minute.

4. Add the onions and sauté for about 2–3 minutes. Add the soy sauce, vinegar, maple syrup, and sesame oil, and bring to a gentle simmer.

5. In the meantime, in a small bowl, dissolve the remaining cornstarch in water. Put the cornstarch batter into the sauce, stirring continuously.

6. Stir in the cooked tofu and cook for about 1 minute. Meanwhile, in a large pan of water, arrange a steamer basket and bring to a boil. Reduce the heat to medium-low.

7. Place the broccoli florets in the steamer basket and steam, covered for about 5–6 minutes. Drain the broccoli and transfer into the skillet of tofu and stir to combine. Serve hot.

Nutrition: Calories 414 Fat 29.7 g Carbs 28.7 g Protein 14 g

18. Veggies & Rice Pilaf

Preparation time: 15 minutes

Cooking time: 60 minutes

Servings: 4

Ingredients:

- 2 tablespoons olive oil
- 2 garlic cloves, minced
- 2 cups fresh mushrooms, sliced
- 1¼ cups brown rice, rinsed
- 2 cups vegetable broth
- Salt and ground black pepper, to taste
- 1 red bell pepper, seeded and chopped
- 4 scallions, chopped
- 1 can red kidney beans, (15-oz) drained & rinsed
- ¼ cup cashews
- 2 tablespoons fresh parsley, chopped

Directions:

1. In a large pan, heat the oil over medium heat and sauté the onion for about 4–5 minutes. Add the garlic and mushrooms and cook about 5–6 minutes.
2. Stir in the rice and cook for about 1–2 minutes, stirring continuously. Stir in the broth, salt, and black pepper, and bring to a boil.

3. Now, adjust the heat to low and simmer, covered for about 35 minutes, stirring occasionally.

4. Add in the bell pepper and beans and cook for about 5–10 minutes or until all the liquid is absorbed. Serve hot with the garnishing of cashews and parsley.

Nutrition: Calories 455 Fat 13.5 g Carbs 69.5 g Protein 16.3 g

19.   Pasta with Bolognese Sauce

Preparation time: 15 minutes

Cooking time: 2 hours

Servings: 6

Ingredients:

Bolognese Sauce:

- 5 tablespoons olive oil, divided
- 3 celery stalks, chopped finely
- 1 medium carrot, peeled and chopped finely
- 1 medium onion, chopped finely
- ¾ cup quinoa, rinsed
- 3 cups fresh mushrooms, chopped
- 2 ounces raw walnuts, chopped
- 4 garlic cloves, chopped
- ¾ teaspoon dried oregano
- ½ teaspoon dried thyme
- ¼ teaspoon dried rosemary
- ¼ teaspoon dried sage
- 1/8 teaspoon red pepper flakes
- 1½ cups vegetable broth
- 1 tablespoon soy sauce
- 1 tablespoon white miso
- 1 teaspoon agar-agar

- 1½ teaspoons paprika
- 1 (14-ounce) can crushed tomatoes
- 1 tablespoon balsamic vinegar
- 4 bay leaves
- 2 tablespoons nutritional yeast
- ¼ cup oat milk
- Salt and ground black pepper, to taste
- ¼ cup fresh basil leaves

Pasta:

- ¾ pound whole-wheat pasta (of your choice)

Directions:

1. Preheat your oven to 300°F. Heat-up 3 tablespoons of the olive oil in a large Dutch oven over medium heat and cook the celery, carrots, and onion for about 10 minutes, stirring frequently.

2. Stir in the quinoa and cook for about 3 minutes. Add the remaining oil, mushrooms, and walnuts, and stir to combine.

3. Now, adjust the heat to medium-high and cook for about 5 minutes. Add the garlic, dried herbs, and red pepper flakes, and cook for about 1–2 minutes.

4. Add the broth and cook for about 5 minutes. Add the soy sauce, miso, agar-agar, and paprika, and stir to combine.

5. Add the tomatoes along with ½ a can of water, vinegar, and bay leaves, and bring to a boil. Remove the Dutch oven from heat and transfer into the oven. Bake, uncovered for about 1½ hours, stirring once after 1 hour.
6. Meanwhile, in a pan of the lightly salted boiling water, cook the pasta for about 8–10 minutes or according to package's instructions. Drain the pasta well.
7. Remove the Dutch oven from oven and stir in the nutritional yeast and oat milk. Divide the pasta onto serving plates and top with Bolognese sauce. Garnish with basil leaves and serve.

Nutrition: Calories 534 Fat 21 g Carbs 29.8 g Protein 20.3 g

20. Spaghetti with Beans Balls

Preparation time: 15 minutes

Cooking time: 35 minutes

Servings: 4

Ingredients:

Beans Balls:

- 1½ tablespoons ground flaxseed
- 4 tablespoons water
- 1½ cups canned chickpeas, drained and rinsed
- ¼ cup whole-wheat breadcrumbs
- 2 tablespoons nutritional yeast
- ½ teaspoon Italian seasoning
- ½ teaspoon onion powder
- ½ teaspoon garlic powder
- Salt, to taste

Pasta:

- ½ pound whole-wheat spaghetti
- 12 ounces sugar-free spaghetti sauce

Directions:

1. Preheat your oven to 425°F. Grease a large baking sheet. For beans balls: In a large bowl, add the ground flax and water and mix well. Set aside for about 5 minutes.

2. In a separate bowl, add the chickpeas and with a potato masher, mash well. Add the flaxseed mixture and remaining ingredients and mix well.

3. Make desired sized balls from the mixture. Arrange the balls onto the prepared baking sheet in a single layer. Bake for approximately 30–35 minutes, flipping once halfway through.

4. Meanwhile, in a pan of the lightly salted boiling water, cook the spaghetti for about 8–10 minutes or according to package's instructions.

5. Drin the spaghetti well. Divide the spaghetti onto serving plates and top with balls and marinara sauce. Serve immediately.

Nutrition: Calories 479 Fat 6.2 g Carbs 89.8 g Protein 19.4 g

21. **Baked Okra and Tomato**

Preparation time: 15 minutes

Cooking time: 1 hour & 15 minutes

Servings: 6

Ingredients:

- ½ cup lima beans, frozen
- 4 tomatoes, chopped
- 8 ounces okra, fresh and washed, stemmed, sliced into ½ inch thick slices
- 1 onion, sliced into rings
- ½ sweet pepper, seeded and sliced thin
- Pinch of crushed red pepper
- Salt to taste

Directions:

1. Preheat your oven to 350 degrees Fahrenheit. Cook lima beans in water accordingly and drain them, take a 2quart casserole tin.
2. Add all listed ingredients to the dish and cover with foil, bake for 45 minutes. Uncover the dish, stir well and bake for 35 minutes more.

3. Give it a final stir, serve and enjoy!

Nutrition: Calories: 55 Fat: 0g Carbohydrates: 12g Protein: 3g

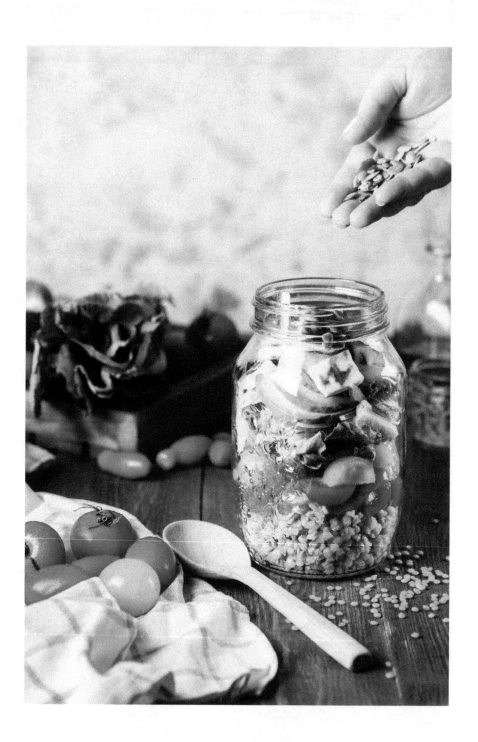

SNACKS

22. Granola Bars with Maple Syrup

Preparation time: 15 minutes

Cooking time: 0 minutes

Servings: 12

Ingredients

- 3/4 cup dates chopped
- 2 tbsp chia seeds soaked
- 3/4 cup rolled oats
- 4 tbsp chopped nuts such macadamia, almond, brazilian...etc.,
- 2 tbsp shredded coconut
- 2 tbsp pumpkin seeds
- 2 tbsp sesame seeds
- 2 tbsp hemp seeds
- 1/2 cup of maple syrup
- 1/4 cup of peanut butter

Directions:

1. Add all ingredients (except maple syrup and peanut butter) into a food processor and pulse just until roughly combined.

2. Add maple syrup and peanut butter and process until all ingredients are combined well. Place baking paper onto a medium baking dish and spread the mixture.

3. Cover with a plastic wrap and press down to make it flat. Chill granola in the fridge for one hour. Cut it into 12 bars and serve.

Nutrition: Calories: 191 Carbs: 27g Fat: 7g Protein: 3g

23. Green Soy Beans Hummus

Preparation time: 15 minutes

Cooking time: 0 minutes

Servings: 6

Ingredients

- 1 1/2 cups frozen green soybeans
- 4 cups of water
- coarse salt to taste
- 1/4 cup sesame paste
- 1/2 tsp grated lemon peel
- 3 tbsp fresh lemon juice
- 2 cloves of garlic crushed
- 1/2 tsp ground cumin
- 1/4 tsp ground coriander
- 4 tbsp extra virgin olive oil
- 1 tbsp fresh parsley leaves chopped
- serving options: sliced cucumber, celery, olives

Directions:

1. In a saucepan, bring to boil 4 cups of water with 2 to 3 pinches of coarse salt. Add in frozen soybeans, and cook for 5 minutes or until tender.

2. Rinse and drain soybeans into a colander. Add soybeans and all remaining ingredients into a food processor.

3. Pulse until smooth and creamy. Taste and adjust salt to taste. Serve with sliced cucumber, celery, olives, bread...etc.

Nutrition : Calories: 150 Carbs: 9g Fat: 7g Protein: 12g

24. Cheese Cucumber Bites

Preparation Time: 10 minutes

Cooking Time: 0 minutes

Servings: 8

Ingredients:

- 4 large cucumbers
- 1 cup raw sunflower seeds
- 1/2 tsp salt
- 2 tbsp. raw red onion, chopped
- 1 handful fresh chives, chopped
- 1 clove fresh garlic, chopped
- 2 tbsp. nutritional yeast
- 2 tbsp. fresh lemon juice
- 1/2 cup water

Directions:

1. Start by blending sunflower seeds with salt in a food processor for 20 seconds. Toss in remaining ingredients except for the cucumber and chives and process until smooth.
2. Slice the cucumber into 1.5-inch-thick rounds. Top each slice with sunflower mixture.

3. Garnish with sumac and chives. Serve.

Nutrition: Calories 211 Fat 25.5 g Carbs 32.4 g Protein 1.4 g

25. <u>**Mango Sticky Rice**</u>

Preparation Time: 15 Minutes

Cooking Time: 20 minutes

Servings: 3

Ingredients:

- ½ cup sugar
- 1 mango, sliced
- 14 ounces coconut milk, canned
- ½ cup basmati rice

Directions:

1. Cook your rice per package instructions, and add half of your sugar. When cooking your rice, substitute half of your water for half of your coconut milk.
2. Boil your remaining coconut milk in a saucepan with your remaining sugar. Boil on high heat until it's thick, and then add in your mango slices.

Nutrition: Calories: 571 Protein: 6 g Fat: 29.6 g Carbs: 77.6 g

26. <u>Green Chips</u>

Preparation time: 15 minutes

Cooking time: 10-20 minutes

Servings: 2

Ingredients:

- 2 or 3 large green leaves or 5 or 6 small leaves of kale, cabbage, collards, orchard, washed, dried, stemmed, and torn into small pieces
- 1 tablespoon olive oil
- 1 tablespoon nutritional yeast (optional)
- 1 teaspoon onion powder (optional)
- Pinch salt

Directions:

1. Preheat the oven to 300°F. Put the greens on a rimmed baking sheet, and sprinkle with the olive oil, nutritional yeast (if using), onion powder (if using), and salt.
2. Massage the spices into the leaves. Spread the leaves out in a single layer so they dry evenly. Bake for 10 to 20 minutes, until the greens are crispy and dry.
3. Remove the greens from the oven, and let them sit for a few minutes to cool before serving.

4. Store in an airtight container, though it's best to bake and enjoy them the same day.

Nutrition: Calories: 93Protein: 2gFat: 7gCarbohydrates: 7g

VEGETABLES

27. Grilled Seitan with Creole Sauce

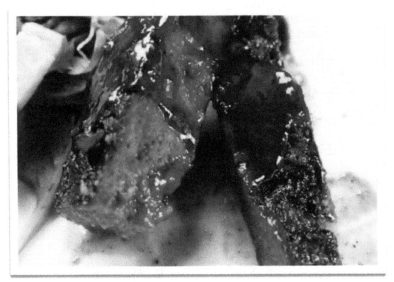

Preparation Time: 10 minutes

Cooking Time: 14 minutes

Servings: 4

Ingredients:

Grilled Seitan Kebabs:

- 4 cups seitan, diced
- 2 medium onions, diced into squares
- 8 bamboo skewers
- 1 can coconut milk

- 2½ tablespoons creole spice
- 2 tablespoons tomato paste
- 2 cloves of garlic

Creole Spice Mix:

- 2 tablespoons paprika
- 12 dried peri chili peppers
- 1 tablespoon salt
- 1 tablespoon freshly ground pepper
- 2 teaspoons dried thyme
- 2 teaspoons dried oregano

Directions:

1. Prepare the creole seasoning by blending all its ingredients and preserve in a sealable jar.
2. Thread seitan and onion on the bamboo skewers in an alternating pattern.
3. On a baking sheet, mix coconut milk with creole seasoning, tomato paste and garlic.
4. Soak the skewers in the milk marinade for 2 hours.
5. Prepare and set up a grill over medium heat.
6. Grill the skewers for 7 minutes per side.

7. Serve.

Nutrition: Calories: 407Total Fat: 42gCarbs: 13gNet Carbs: 6g Fiber: 1gProtein: 4g

28. Green Beans Gremolata

Preparation Time: 15 minutes

Cooking Time: 5 minutes

Serving: 6

Ingredients:

- 1-pound fresh green beans
- 3 garlic cloves, minced
- Zest of 2 oranges
- 3 tablespoons minced fresh parsley
- 2 tablespoons pine nuts
- 3 tablespoons olive oil
- Sea salt
- Freshly ground black pepper

Direction:

1. Boil water over high heat. Cook green beans for 3 minutes. Drain r and rinse with cold water to stop the cooking.

2. Blend garlic, orange zest, and parsley.

3. In a huge sauté pan over medium-high heat, toast the pine nuts in the dry, hot pan for 3 minutes. Remove from the pan and set aside.

4. Cook olive oil in the same pan until it shimmers. Add the beans and cook, -stirring frequently, until heated

through, about 2 minutes. Take pan away from the heat and add the parsley mixture and pine nuts. Season with salt and pepper. Serve immediately.

Nutrition: 98 Calories 2g Fiber 3g Protein

SALAD

29. Tempeh "Chicken" Salad

Preparation Time: 10 minutes

Cooking Time: 0 minutes

Servings: 2

Ingredients:

- 4 tablespoons light mayonnaise
- 2 scallions, sliced
- Pepper to taste
- 4 cups mixed salad greens
- 4 teaspoons white miso
- 2 tablespoons chopped fresh dill
- 1 ½ cups crumbled tempeh
- 1 cup sliced grape tomatoes

Directions:

To make dressing:

1. Add mayonnaise, scallions, miso, dill and pepper into a bowl and whisk well.
2. Add tempeh and fold gently.

To serve:

3. Divide the greens into 4 plates. Divide the tempeh among the plates. Top with tomatoes and serve.

Nutrition: Calories 452Total Fat 24.5gSaturated Fat 4.4gCholesterol 8mgSodium 733mgTotal Carbohydrate 37.2gDietary Fiber 2.6gTotal Sugars 5.3gProtein 29.9gVitamin D 0mcgCalcium 261mgIron 8mgPotassium 1377mg

30. **Spinach & Dill Pasta Salad**

Preparation Time: 5 minutes

Cooking Time: 0 minutes

Servings: 4

Ingredients:

For salad:

- 3 cups cooked whole-wheat fusilli
- 2 cups cherry tomatoes, halved
- ½ cup vegan cheese, shredded
- 4 cups spinach, chopped
- 2 cups edamame, thawed
- 1 large red onion, finely chopped

For dressing:

- 2 tablespoons white wine vinegar
- ½ teaspoon dried dill
- 2 tablespoons extra-virgin olive oil
- Salt to taste
- Pepper to taste

Directions:

To make dressing:

1. Add all the ingredients for dressing into a bowl and whisk well. Set aside for a while for the flavors to set in.

To make salad:

2. Add all the ingredients of the salad in a bowl. Toss well.
3. Drizzle dressing on top. Toss well.
4. Divide into 4 plates and serve.

Nutrition: Calories 684Total Fat 33.6gSaturated Fat 4.6g Cholesterol 4mgSodium 632mgTotal Carbohydrate 69.5gDietary Fiber 12gTotal Sugars 6.4gProtein 31.7gVitamin D 0mcgCalcium 368mgIron 8mgPotassium 1241mg

GRAINS

31. Vinegary Black Beans

Preparation Time: 10 minutes

Cooking Time: 2 hours

Servings: 8

Ingredients:

- 1 pound (454 g) black beans, soaked overnight and drained
- 10½ cups water, divided
- 1 green bell pepper, cut in half
- 1 onion, finely chopped
- 1 green bell pepper, finely chopped
- 4 cloves garlic, pressed
- 1 tablespoon maple syrup (optional)
- 1 tablespoon Mrs. Dash seasoning
- 1 bay leaf
- ¼ teaspoon dried oregano
- 2 tablespoons cider vinegar

Directions:

1. Place the beans, 10 cups of the water, and green bell pepper in a large pot. Cook over medium heat for

about 45 minutes, or until the green pepper is tendered. Remove the green pepper and discard.

2. Meanwhile, in a different pot, combine the onion, chopped green pepper, garlic and the remaining ½ cup of the water. Sauté for 15 to 20 minutes, or until soft.

3. Add 1 cup of the cooked beans to the pot with vegetables. Mash the beans and vegetables with a potato masher. Add to the pot with the beans, maple syrup (if desired), Mrs. Dash, bay leaf and oregano. Cover and cook over low heat for 1 hour.

4. Drizzle in the vinegar and continue to cook for another hour.

5. Serve warm.

Nutrition: calories: 226 fat: 0.9g carbs: 42.7g protein: 12.9g fiber: 9.9g

32. **Spiced Lentil Burgers**

Preparation Time: 10 minutes

Cooking Time: 43 minutes

Servings: 4

Ingredients:

- ¼ cup minced onion
- 1 clove garlic, minced
- 2 tablespoons water
- 1 cup chopped boiled potatoes
- 1 cup cooked lentils
- 2 tablespoons minced fresh parsley
- 1 teaspoon onion powder
- 1 teaspoon minced fresh basil
- 1 teaspoon dried dill
- 1 teaspoon paprika

Directions:

1. Preheat the oven to 350°F (180°C).
2. In a pot, sauté the onion and garlic in the water for about 3 minutes, or until soft.
3. Combine the lentils and potatoes in a large bowl and mash together well. Add the cooked onion and garlic and the remaining ingredients to the lentil-potato mixture and stir until well combined.

4. Form the mixture into four patties and place on a nonstick baking sheet. Bake in the oven for 20 minutes. Turnover and bake for an additional 20 minutes.
5. Serve hot.

Nutrition: calories: 101fat: 0.4gcarbs: 19.9gprotein: 5.5gfiber: 5.3g

LEGUMES

33. Middle Eastern Chickpea Stew

Preparation Time: 10 minutes

Cooking Time: 10 minutes

Servings: 4

Ingredients:

- 1 onion, chopped
- 1 chili pepper, chopped
- 2 garlic cloves, chopped
- 1 teaspoon mustard seeds
- 1 teaspoon coriander seeds
- 1 bay leaf
- 1/2 cup tomato puree
- 2 tablespoons olive oil
- 1 celery with leaves, chopped
- 2 medium carrots, trimmed and chopped
- 2 cups vegetable broth
- 1 teaspoon ground cumin
- 1 small-sized cinnamon stick
- 16 ounces canned chickpeas, drained
- 2 cups Swiss chard, torn into pieces

Directions

1. In your blender or food processor, blend the onion, chili pepper, garlic, mustard seeds, coriander seeds, bay leaf and tomato puree into a paste.

2. In a stockpot, heat the olive oil until sizzling. Now, cook the celery and carrots for about 3 minutes or until they've softened. Add in the paste and continue to cook for a further 2 minutes.

3. Then, add vegetable broth, cumin, cinnamon and chickpeas; bring it to a gentle boil.

4. Turn the heat to simmer and let it cook for 6 minutes; fold in Swiss chard and continue to cook for 4 to 5 minutes more or until the leaves wilt. Serve hot and enjoy!

Nutrition: Calories: 305; Fat: 11.2g; Carbs: 38.6g; Protein: 12.7g

34. __Lentil and Tomato Dip__

Preparation Time: 10 minutes

Cooking Time: 10 minutes

Servings: 4

Ingredients:

- 16 ounces' lentils, boiled and drained
- 4 tablespoons sun-dried tomatoes, chopped
- 1 cup tomato paste
- 4 tablespoons tahini
- 1 teaspoon stone-ground mustard
- 1 teaspoon ground cumin
- 1/4 teaspoon ground bay leaf
- 1 teaspoon red pepper flakes
- Sea salt and ground black pepper, to taste

Directions

1. Blitz all the ingredients in your blender or food processor until your desired consistency is reached.
2. Place in your refrigerator until ready to serve.
3. Serve with toasted pita wedges or vegetable sticks. Enjoy!

Nutrition: Calories: 144; Fat: 4.5g; Carbs: 20.2g; Protein: 8.1g

BREAD & PIZZA

35. Buttermilk Biscuits

Preparation Time: 15 Minutes

Cooking Time: 15 Minutes

Servings: 8

Ingredients:

- 1 cup plant-based milk
- 1 tablespoon apple cider vinegar
- 2 cups unbleached all-purpose flour, plus more for cutting out the biscuits
- 1 tablespoon baking powder
- 1/2 teaspoon baking soda
- 1/2 teaspoon salt
- 1 tablespoon cane sugar
- 4 tablespoons (1/2 stick) Earth Balance vegan butter, cold

Directions:

1. Preheat the oven to 450-degree F and line a baking pan with parchment paper.
2. In a small bowl, mix the milk and vinegar and allow to curdle, usually no more than 5 minutes.

3. In a medium mixing bowl, whisk together the flour, baking powder, baking soda, salt, and sugar.

4. Add the cold butter and use your fingers or a pastry cutter to combine until only small pieces remain and the mixture looks grainy, like sand. Work fast so the butter doesn't get too soft.

5. Make a well in the dry Ingredients, and use a wooden spoon to stir gently while pouring in the milk mixture 1/4 cup at a time. Stir until well combined.

6. Sprinkle flour on a clean surface and dump the dough onto it. Dust the top of the dough with flour. Gently flatten the dough with your hands until it is about 1 inch thick, then dip a coffee mug rim into the flour to coat it and use it to cut out the biscuits.

7. Place the cut biscuits on the lined baking pan, and bake for 6 minutes, then turn and bake another 6 minutes or until the tops and edges turn golden brown.

Nutrition: Calories 115, Carbs 2.5g, Fat 10.5g, Protein 4.7g

36. __Keto Cheese Bread__

Preparation time: 9 minutes

Cooking time: 25 minutes

Servings: 6

Ingredients:

- 1 teaspoon Baking Powder
- 1/4 teaspoon Salt
- 1/3 cup Milk
- 1 cup Almond Flour
- 2 large Whole Eggs
- 1/3 cup Cream Cheese, softened
- 1/2 cup Grated Parmesan

Directions:

1. Preheat oven to 350-degree F.
2. Whisk together almond flour, baking powder, and salt in a bowl.
3. In a separate, bowl beat eggs and add cream cheese. Gradually stir in the milk.
4. Stir the wet mixture into the dry Ingredients.
5. Fold in the grated parmesan.
6. Coat a 6-hole muffin tin with non-stick spray.

7. Divide the batter into the pan and bake for 25 minutes.

Nutrition: Calories 203 Carbohydrates 6 g Fats 16 g Protein 9 g

SOUP AND STEW

37. Avocado Mint Soup

Preparation Time: 10 minutes

Cooking Time: 10 minutes

Servings: 2

Ingredients:

- 1 medium avocado, peeled, pitted, and cut into pieces
- 1 cup coconut milk
- 2 romaine lettuce leaves
- 20 fresh mint leaves
- 1 tbsp fresh lime juice
- 1/8 tsp salt

Directions:

1. Add all ingredients into the blender and blend until smooth. Soup should be thick not as a puree.
2. Pour into the serving bowls and place in the refrigerator for 10 minutes.
3. Stir well and serve chilled.

Nutrition: Calories: 377 kcalFat: 14.9g Carbs: 60.7g

Protein: 6.4g

38. Creamy Squash Soup

Preparation Time: 10 minutes

Cooking Time: 25 minutes

Servings: 8

Ingredients:

- 3 cups butternut squash, chopped
- 1 ½ cups unsweetened coconut milk
- 1 tbsp coconut oil
- 1 tsp dried onion flakes
- 1 tbsp curry powder
- 4 cups water
- 1 garlic clove
- 1 tsp kosher salt

Directions:

1. Add squash, coconut oil, onion flakes, curry powder, water, garlic, and salt into a large saucepan. Bring to boil over high heat.
2. Turn heat to medium and simmer for 20 minutes.
3. Puree the soup using a blender until smooth. Return soup to the saucepan and stir in coconut milk and cook for 2 minutes.

4. Stir well and serve hot.

Nutrition: Calories: 271 kcalFat: 3.7g Carbs: 54g Protein:6.5g

SAUCES, DRESSINGS & DIP

39. Pineapple Mint Salsa

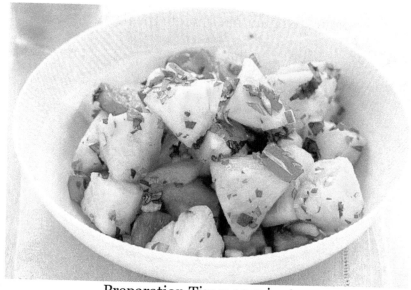

Preparation Time: 10 minutes

Cooking Time: 0 minutes

Servings: 3

Ingredients:

- 1 pound (454 g) fresh pineapple, finely diced and juices reserved
- 1 bunch mint, leaves only, chopped
- 1 minced jalapeño, (optional)
- 1 white or red onion, finely diced
- Salt, to taste (optional)

Directions:

1. In a medium bowl, mix the pineapple with its juice, mint, jalapeño (if desired), and onion, and whisk well. Season with salt to taste, if desired.

2. Refrigerate in an airtight container for at least 2 hours to better incorporate the flavors.

Nutrition: calories: 58fat: 0.1g carbs: 13.7g protein: 0.5g fiber: 1.0g

40. <u>Keto Salsa Verde</u>

Preparation time: 10 minutes

Cooking time: 5 minutes

Servings: 5

Ingredients:

- 4 tablespoons fresh cilantro, finely chopped
- 1/4 cup fresh parsley, finely chopped
- 2 garlic cloves, grated
- 2 teaspoon lemon juice
- 3/4 cup of olive oil
- 2 tablespoon small capers
- 1 teaspoon of salt
- 1/2 teaspoon black pepper

Directions:

1. Add all **Ingredients:** to a large mixing bowl. Can be mixed with by hand or with an immersion blender. Mix until desired consistency is achieved.

2. Can be served over burgers, sandwiches, salads and more.

3. Can be stored in the refrigerator for up to 5 days or for longer in the freezer.

Nutrition: Total fat: 25.3g Cholesterol: 0mg Sodium: 475mg Protein: 0.2g

APPETIZER

41. Seeded Crackers

Preparation Time: 1 hour

Cooking Time: 10 minutes

Servings: 36 crackers

Ingredients:

- ½ cup pumpkin seeds
- ½ cup sunflower seeds
- ¼ cup sesame seeds
- ¼ cup chia seeds
- ¾ cup water
- ¾ teaspoon salt
- 1 teaspoon rosemary
- 1 teaspoon onion powder

Directions:

1. Preheat oven to 350°F. Set aside two large pieces of parchment paper. Combine all ingredients in a large bowl. Set aside to rest for 15 minutes.
2. Oil one side of each of the two sheets of parchment paper to avoid sticking in the next step.

3. Place the dough between the two pieces of parchment paper. Roll-out your dough thin using a rolling pin (roll to approximately 10 x 14-inch rectangle).

4. Slide the rolled-out dough onto a baker's half sheet. Bake for 20 minutes. Remove from oven and cut into large pieces. Flip each piece over when finished. Bake for an additional 14 minutes. Serve.

Nutrition: Calories 26 Fat 2 gProtein 1 gCarbs 2 g

42. **Banana Bites**

Preparation Time: 15 minutes

Cooking Time: 15 minutes

Servings: 4

Ingredients:

- 2 bananas
- ½ cup vegan chocolate, melted
- 1 cup roasted pistachios, in pieces or finely crushed

Directions:

1. Set aside a parchment-lined baking sheet. Peel the bananas and stick a toothpick in both ends to make the next step easier.
2. Dip and fully coat the bananas in the melted chocolate. Set onto the parchment paper.
3. If using whole pistachios, place the nuts into a food processor and pulse until fine. Leave some pistachios intact.
4. Sprinkle the pistachios on top of the banana. Freeze the bananas to set the chocolate and pistachios for 5 minutes.
5. Remove the bananas and cut into bites. Return to the freezer in a glass container.

6. When ready to consume, remove bananas from the freezer and thaw for 10 minutes to soften.

Nutrition: Calories 273Fat 14 gProtein 6 gCarbs 37 g

43. <u>Plantain Chips</u>

Cooking Time: 15 minutes

Preparation Time: 35 minutes

Servings: 4

Ingredients:

- 2 green (slightly yellow) plantains, washed and peeled
- ½ tablespoon onion powder
- ½ tablespoon paprika
- ½ teaspoon salt
- 1½ tablespoon avocado oil

Directions:

1. Preheat the oven to 350°F. Cut the plantains into very thin slices using a sharp knife. Place the slices into a medium mixing bowl.
2. In a small bowl, whisk together all the spices and avocado oil. Pour mixture into the bowl containing the plantains. Mix until well incorporated.
3. Place plantains onto a large non-stick baking sheet. Bake for 20 minutes. Remove and let cool before serving.

Nutrition: Calories 200Fat 10 gProtein 2 gCarbs 30 g

SMOOTHIES AND JUICES

44. **Berry and Yogurt Smoothie**

Preparation time: 5 minutes

Cooking time: 0 minute

Servings: 2

Ingredients:

- 2 small bananas
- 3 cups frozen mixed berries
- 1 ½ cup cashew yogurt
- 1/2 teaspoon vanilla extract, unsweetened
- 1/2 cup almond milk, unsweetened

Directions:

1. Place all the ingredients in the order in a food processor or blender and then pulse for 2 to 3 minutes at high speed until smooth.
2. Pour the smoothie into two glasses and then serve.

Nutrition Value: Calories: 326 Cal Fat: 6.5 g Carbs: 65.6 g Protein: 8 g Fiber: 8.4 g

45. <u>Chocolate and Cherry Smoothie</u>

Preparation time: 5 minutes

Cooking time: 0 minute

Servings: 2

Ingredients:

- 4 cups frozen cherries
- 2 tablespoons cocoa powder
- 1 scoop of protein powder
- 1 teaspoon maple syrup
- 2 cups almond milk, unsweetened

Directions:

1. Place all the ingredients in the order in a food processor or blender and then pulse for 2 to 3 minutes at high speed until smooth.
2. Pour the smoothie into two glasses and then serve.

Nutrition: Calories: 324 Cal Fat: 5 g Carbs: 75.1 g Protein: 7.2 g Fiber: 11.3 g

DESSERTS

46. **Coconut and Pineapple Pudding**

Preparation time: 15 minutes

Cooking time: 30 minutes

Servings: 2

Ingredients:

- 2 tablespoons ground flaxseeds
- 2 cups unsweetened almond milk
- 1 tablespoon maple syrup
- ¼ cup chia seeds
- 1 teaspoon vanilla extract
- 2 tablespoons shredded, unsweetened coconut
- 1 Medjool date, pitted and chopped
- 2 cups sliced pineapple

Directions:

1. Put the flaxseeds, almond milk, maple syrup, chia seeds, and vanilla extract in a bowl. Stir to mix well.
2. Put the bowl in the refrigerator within 20 minutes, then remove from the refrigerator and stir again. Place the bowl back to the refrigerator for 30 minutes or overnight to make the pudding.

3. Mix in the coconut, and spread the date and pineapple on top before serving.

Nutrition: Calories: 513 Fat: 22.9g Carbs: 66.4g Protein: 16.2g

47. **<u>Sweet Potato Toast with Blueberries</u>**

Preparation time: 15 minutes

Cooking time: 30 minutes

Servings: 10 slices

Ingredients:

- 1 large sweet potato, rinsed and cut into 10 slices
- 20 blueberries
- 2 tablespoons almond butter

Directions:

1. Warm your oven to 350°F. Put a wire rack on your baking sheet. Arrange the sweet potato slices on the wire rack, then cook in the preheated oven for 15 or until soft.
2. Flip the sweet potato slices for every 5 minutes to make sure evenly cooked. Then toast immediately or store in the refrigerator.
3. To make the sweet potato toast, put the cooked sweet potato slices in a toaster in batches and toast over medium for 15 minutes or until crispy and golden brown. Serve the toast with blueberries and almond butter.

Nutrition: Calories: 374 Fat: 18.1g Carbs: 47.2g Protein: 10.5g

48. No-Bake Green Energy Super Bars

Preparation time: 15 minutes

Cooking time: 0 minutes

Servings: 36 bars

Ingredients:

- 1½ cups pitted dates, soaked in hot water for 5 minutes and drained
- ½ cup roasted, unsalted cashews
- ½ cup raw sunflower seeds
- 2 tablespoons spirulina powder
- ¼ cup carob
- 2 tablespoons unsweetened shredded coconut
- Pinch of salt, optional

Directions:

1. Put the dates in your blender then process to make the date paste. Add the cashews, sunflower seeds, spirulina powder, and carob. Pulse until dough-like and thick.
2. Put the batter in a baking dish lined using parchment paper, then sprinkle with coconut and salt (if desired).
3. Let stand for 5 minutes, then pull the parchment paper with the mixture out of the container and cut the mixture into 36 bars.

4. Serve immediately.

Nutrition: Calories: 1729 Fat: 79.0g Carbs: 231.0g Protein: 33.0g

49. <u>Strawberry Sushi</u>

Preparation time: 15 minutes

Cooking time: 25 minutes

Servings: 24 sushi

Ingredients:

- 3 cups cooked white sushi rice
- 3 tablespoons fresh lemon juice
- ½ teaspoon vanilla extract
- ½ cup maple sugar
- 2 cups strawberries, hulled and quartered
- 3 tablespoons chia seeds
- Salt, to taste (optional)

Directions:

1. Combine the cooked sushi rice, lemon juice, vanilla extract, and maple sugar in a large bowl. Stir to mix well.

2. Wrap a sushi mat with plastic wrap, then arrange 1 cup of rice on top and press into ½-inch thick.

3. Arrange a row of strawberries on the rice and leave a 1-inch gap from the bottom side. Sprinkle with 1 teaspoon of chia seeds.

4. Use the plastic wrap and sushi mat to help to roll the rice into a cylinder. When you roll, pull the plastic wrap

and sushi mat away from the rice at the same time. Repeat with the remaining rice and chia seeds.

5. Sprinkle the rolls with salt, if desired. Let stand for 5 minutes and slice each roll into 8 sushi. Serve immediately.

Nutrition: Calories: 295 Carbs: 55g Fat: 6g Protein: 5g

50. Pecan, Coconut, and Chocolate Bars

Preparation time: 15 minutes

Cooking time: 10 minutes

Servings: 8 bars

Ingredients:

- 1 cup pitted dates, soaked/dipped in hot water within 10 minutes and drained
- ¼ cup maple syrup
- 1½ cups rolled oats
- 1/3 cup plus ¼ cup chopped pecans
- 1/3 cup unsweetened shredded coconut
- 1/3 cup mini chocolate chips

Directions:

1. Preheat the oven to 300°F. Line a baking dish with parchment paper. Put the dates in your blender then process to make the date paste, then combine the date paste with maple syrup in a bowl.
2. Put ½ cup of the oats and ¼ cup of the pecans in the blender and process to grind. Mix them in the bowl of date mixture. Stir in the remaining oats and pecans, coconut, and chocolate chips.
3. Pour the mixture in the baking dish and bake in the preheated oven for 10 minutes or until lightly browned.

4. Remove the baking dish from the oven and slice the chunk into 8 bars. Serve immediately.

Nutrition: Calories: 270 Carbs: 41g Fat: 10g Protein: 6g

CPSIA information can be obtained
at www.ICGtesting.com
Printed in the USA
LVHW081911250421
685408LV00003B/44